MW00626346

Printed in Canada

First Edition, 2019

www.natalist.com

Thank you to everyone who contributed to make this book possible: Austin Ledzian, Helen Rice, & Luisa Lacsamana

Medicine is a constantly evolving field. As new research and clinical experience broaden our knowledge, changes in standard of care treatment may become apparent or appropriate. It is the responsibility of the treating physician or provider, relying on their experience and knowledge, to determine the best treatment for each individual patient. Neither the authors nor Natalist assume any liability for any injury and/or damage to persons or property arising from this publication.

Conception 101

Everything you need to know
from concept to conception

Table of Contents

Intro

About 90% of couples will get pregnant naturally in the first year of trying.[1] We really hope you're part of the lucky 90%; but if you're not, hang in there. There are many paths to parenthood. The three of us are a representative mix of experiences. Most importantly, we are all now proud moms.

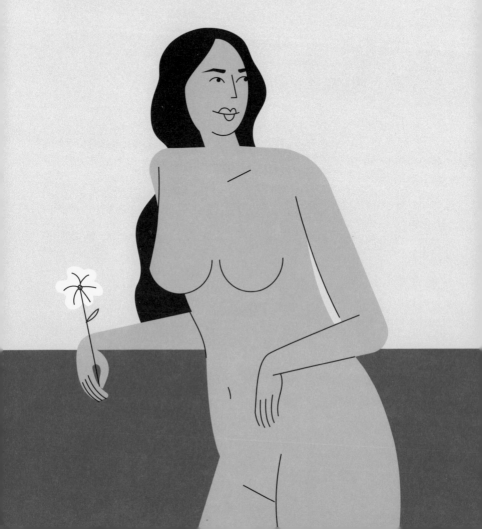

Thinking back to sex ed, we're mostly taught how not to get pregnant—so when it comes time to actually have a baby, there's a lot of ground to cover. How are you supposed to get the info you need, and none of the BS you don't?

We wrote this book to give you the latest, evidence-backed information on how to make that happen. This guide will help you prepare your body, your mind, and your life to have a baby. We'll talk through what a woman's period is actually doing (besides causing those painful cramps), how men and women can support their fertility with lifestyle changes, and what all future parents need to know when they go to the doctor's office for their baby-planning appointment.

The first thing you should know? The experience of getting pregnant and having a baby is different for everyone—there are many shades of normal. Think of this as an opportunity to really get to know your body in all its glory. We're here to talk through the practical stuff— how to figure out the fertile window, prepare for pregnancy, and increase the chances of getting pregnant—while celebrating and acknowledging that this part of life can run a spectrum of emotions: excitement and happiness to frustration and sadness.

This book is geared towards heterosexual, partnered couples trying to get pregnant. When referring to people, we use the terms "woman" and "man" in place of "female" and "male" —the medical terms specifying a person's assigned sex at birth. We recognize that your biology doesn't dictate your gender and not all of our readers will fall into these two categories.

Dr. Nazaneen Homaifar
Chief Medical Advisor

Dr. Elizabeth Kane
Chief Scientific Officer

Halle Tecco
Chief Executive Officer

The Birds and the Bees

Remember sex ed in middle school with the cryptic video of a sperm swimming to an egg, fertilizing it, and immediately creating an embryo? Hot damn, that was quick! The message was always, "Have sex and BOOM. Pregnant!" Well, for the vast majority it's not quite that easy. Fast forward 10-20 years to when you're trying to get pregnant on purpose. All of the sudden, the questions start brewing, "Wait, how exactly does sperm get to the egg?" and "Why is this not happening as fast as I thought it would?" Don't worry, after a quick review of the biological basics, the initial "how" of getting pregnant won't seem so elusive.

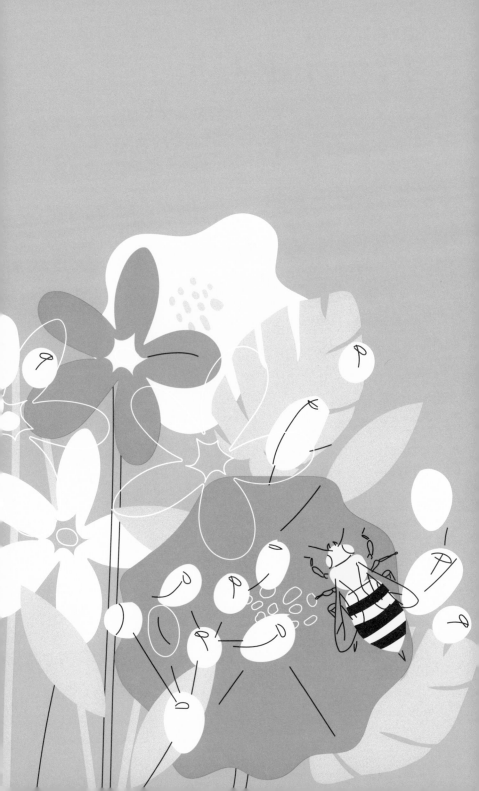

Figure 1

The Female Reproductive System

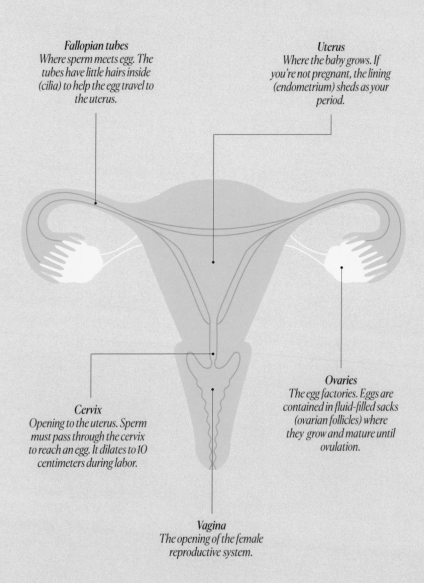

Fallopian tubes
Where sperm meets egg. The tubes have little hairs inside (cilia) to help the egg travel to the uterus.

Uterus
Where the baby grows. If you're not pregnant, the lining (endometrium) sheds as your period.

Cervix
Opening to the uterus. Sperm must pass through the cervix to reach an egg. It dilates to 10 centimeters during labor.

Ovaries
The egg factories. Eggs are contained in fluid-filled sacks (ovarian follicles) where they grow and mature until ovulation.

Vagina
The opening of the female reproductive system.

The Female Reproductive System

Did you know most women are born with two million eggs in their ovaries—their entire lifetime supply? These eggs are immature, and most of them will never have the chance to become fertilized. This may make it seem like you have two million chances to conceive, but it's actually far less. Only a tiny fraction of your eggs will mature (one in 4,000) and have a chance to undergo fertilization and grow.[2]

The maturation process of your eggs is kick-started during puberty, when a flood of hormones pushes them, and a host of other biological processes, down the hill of adulthood. Taking center stage (besides the general awkwardness of adolescence) is the start of menstruation, also known as your period. This marks the beginning of your reproductive window, which lasts until menopause (the time at which you run out of eggs).

Behold, Figure 2: the menstrual cycle, a complex system with a few key players. First, let's get into the hormones that pull most of the strings. Two of them are produced in the brain: follicle stimulating hormone (FSH) and luteinizing hormone (LH), and two of them are produced in the ovaries: progesterone and estrogen. They each play a critical part in a woman's period.

On day one of your period, women are in what's called the *follicular phase* of their cycle. It's good to keep track of this moment on a calendar when trying to conceive—doctors will likely ask about a woman's last menstrual cycle, and this is the date they're looking for. This phase in the cycle is named for the *ovarian follicle*, a fluid-filled sac in the ovary that contains an egg and its associated support cells.

What happens next is a cascade of activity: FSH tells the ovaries to begin to mature the tiny eggs within the follicles. The maturation and growth of these eggs is called oogenesis. As the ovarian follicles grow, they make more estrogen, signaling to the uterus to thicken its lining (the endometrium) and telling the brain to coordinate ovulation.

The estrogen-flooded brain releases a spike of LH—the LH surge—to tell one of the ovaries to release an egg. The ovaries usually take turns doing this, though the work isn't always evenly split. The LH surge is also a convenient marker of the fertile window, the days when a woman is most likely to conceive. We'll go into more

Figure 2

The Menstrual Cycle and its Key Hormonal Regulators

Changes that occur in hormone levels, ovarian follicle development, and basal body temperature for a 28-day menstrual cycle. Ovulation occurs on day 14, and the fertile window is indicated in pink from days 9-14. The first half of the cycle is the follicular phase, the second half is the luteal phase.

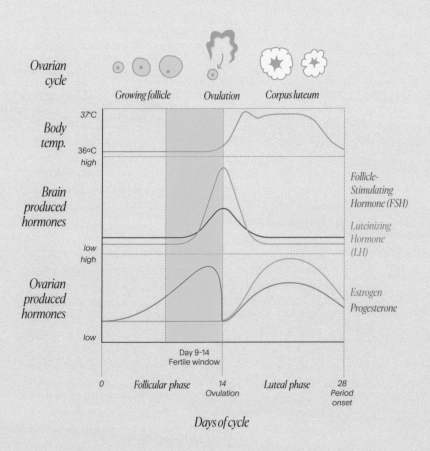

detail about how to find your fertile window and when exactly it is in the next section.

It's time for the big event: ovulation. A now-mature egg breaks out of its ovarian follicle and through the ovarian wall, journeying down the fallopian tube where it'll wait for sperm to fertilize it (or not). Meanwhile, the ovarian follicle transforms into a little hormone factory called the *corpus luteum*, which starts producing lots of progesterone. Progesterone signals to the uterus to thicken its lining, turning it into a cozy home where a fertilized embryo would thrive. This is called the *luteal phase* of your cycle.

If the egg in the fallopian tube meets a sperm, then fertilization occurs and it is transformed into an embryo! But wait—pregnancy is not ensured just yet. The embryo must journey down the fallopian tube into the uterus, and find a spot to call home where it will implant (Figure 3). This whole journey takes about nine days from ovulation.[3] Only after implantation is a pregnancy detectable, hence the nail-biting two-week wait (or TWW for those familiar with trying-to-conceive lingo) between ovulation and when you can test for pregnancy.

If sperm doesn't meet egg, then a period ensues as usual. In the absence of fertilization and implantation, the corpus luteum will stop producing progesterone and break down. No more progesterone means no more thick uterine lining. In response to the withdrawal of estrogen and progesterone in the system, the lining sheds off and leaves the system as your period. This whole cycle (from initial FSH release to period onset) lasts on average from 28 to 35 days, with approximately 14 to 21 days in the follicular phase and 14 days in the luteal phase.

Every cycle, the uterus goes through this laborious process to prepare the perfect environment for an embryo. Despite the discomfort this cycle can bring, the female body and its biological prowess is quite miraculous.

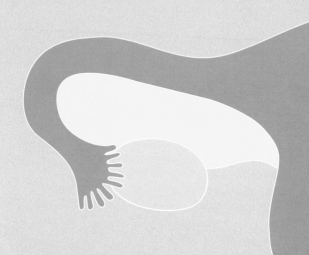

Figure 3

From Ovulation to Implantation

The process of fertilization begins when an ovarian follicle matures (1-3) and releases an egg (4, ovulation). The follicle transforms into a corpus luteum (5). The egg can then be fertilized in the fallopian tube (6). The genetic material of the sperm and egg combine (7, 8) and cell division begins to start (9). The embryo will grow and migrate down the fallopian tube and into the uterus (10-13) until the 7th to 10th day post-fertilization, when it will implant itself into the uterine wall (14).

Adapted from Jones and Lopez, 2006.[2]

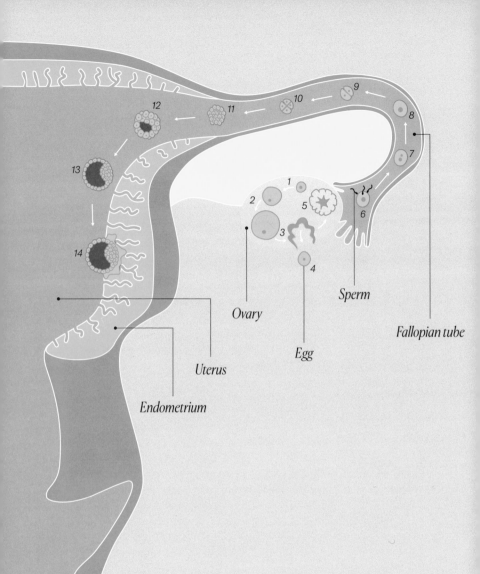

Fallopian tube

Sperm

Ovary

Egg

Uterus

Endometrium

The Fertile Window

Now we've reviewed the basics. Ejaculation releases sperm; they swim up to meet the egg in the fallopian tube; one triumphant sperm burrows into the egg to fertilize it; the fertilized egg journeys down the fallopian tube and implants in the uterine wall and then—pregnancy! But what actually goes down when the magic happens? And how do you time sex to make sure sperm is waiting to fertilize the egg when it is released?

All days are not equal when it comes to making a baby (Figure 4). A woman is most likely to conceive during her *fertile window*—a six day period that starts five days before ovulation and ends on the day of ovulation. The length of the fertile window is set by two things:

1. *The time that sperm can survive in the fallopian tubes.* Amazingly, sperm can live inside the fallopian tubes for five to six days.[5] This means that if you have sex five days before you ovulate, sperm could survive and stick around to fertilize an embryo five days later when you ovulate. Sperm are amazingly resilient.

2. *The time that an egg can survive after ovulation.* Eggs can only survive for about a day after ovulation, so the fertile window ends when this window closes.

So how do you find your fertile window and time sex optimally? There are subtle changes in a woman's body during her fertile window that can be detected (like cervical mucus and basal body temperature) and tools you can use to detect the LH surge that initiates ovulation (ovulation tests). We'll tell you more about these in the next chapters. It's also likely that a woman will ovulate right in the middle of her cycle; so if her cycle is 28 days long, that means on average she would most likely ovulate on day 14. Research says it's best to have sex every day or every other day during the fertile window to maximize chances for pregnancy.[4]

All this talk about timed intercourse and the fertile window can turn sex into an algorithm, which isn't a turn-on for most of us. Emotions and mood matter, and having sex isn't as simple as just deciding to do it. But having sex in a new context can bring you closer with your partner. Acknowledge the good and the bad, talk about how you want to approach the process, and figure out how to cope with the potential stress and disappointment if it doesn't work the first few times around.

Figure 4

Probability of Pregnancy on Each Day of the Menstrual Cycle

This graph shows the probability of pregnancy from a single act of sex each day of the menstrual cycle. It demonstrates that a woman is most likely to conceive during the fertile window.

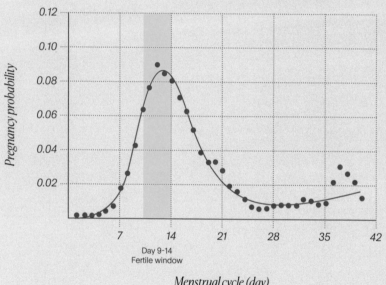

Adapted from Fertil Steril, 2008.[4]

The Male Reproductive System

We've talked about how to use a uterus for good (having a baby!) instead of evil (period cramps). But what about the other half of the equation—the male reproductive system?

Sperm (male sex cells) are produced and housed in the testes (Figure 5). Men start making sperm in puberty (unlike women, who are born with their lifetime supply of eggs) and continue throughout their adult life, without going through a male equivalent of menopause (although sperm quality does decrease with age). Individual sperm cells take a long time to develop—at least two months—and it takes about three months for a sperm to go from the beginnings of formation to release.[2]

What about the numbers—how many sperm do men make throughout their life? It's pretty staggering. The average number of sperm produced from puberty until death is roughly 1,500 per second *(yes per second!).*[2] That's a lot of sperm and would require comically large testes if they were all housed at once.

For men, the hormone that plays the biggest role in baby-making is testosterone. Without adequate testosterone, men are infertile. Women actually also have testosterone, but it's present in lower levels, and mainly promotes bone strength and muscle mass—as it does for men, too.

While we're on the topic of shared hormones: a man's body also produces LH (which initiates the production of testosterone), FSH (which promotes the growth of the testes, rather than ovaries), and estrogen (which men have much less of than women—but it still impacts sex drive, among other things).

A teaspoon of ejaculated semen contains roughly 200 million sperm.[2]

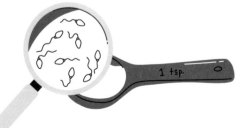

Figure 5

The Male Reproductive System

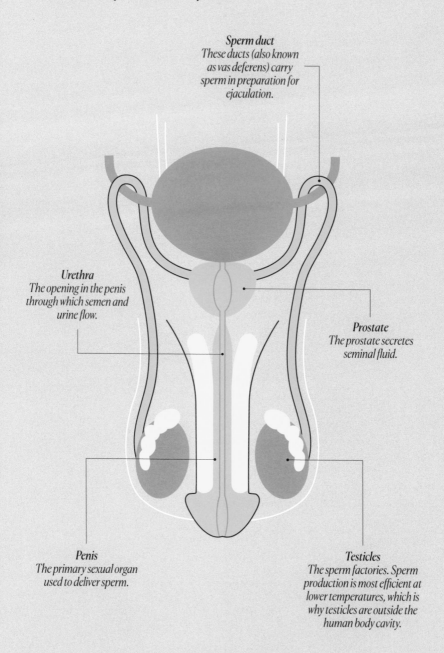

Sperm duct
These ducts (also known as vas deferens) carry sperm in preparation for ejaculation.

Urethra
The opening in the penis through which semen and urine flow.

Prostate
The prostate secretes seminal fluid.

Penis
The primary sexual organ used to deliver sperm.

Testicles
The sperm factories. Sperm production is most efficient at lower temperatures, which is why testicles are outside the human body cavity.

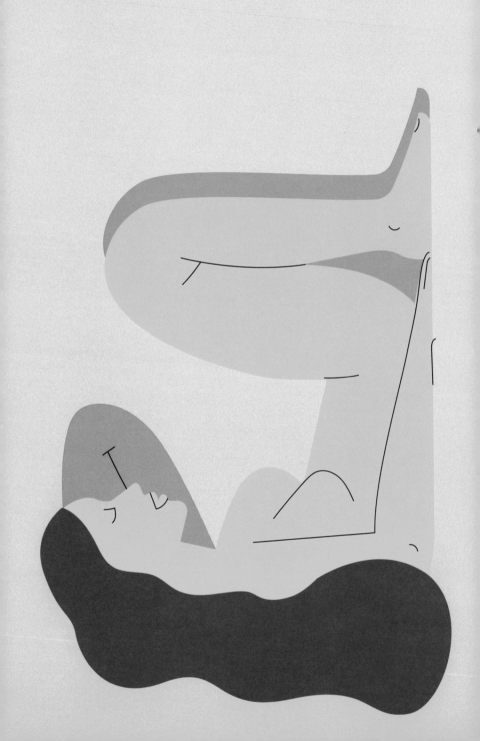

Fertility Myths

There is a lot of junk science and misinformation about conception, fertility, and pregnancy out there. Let's take a moment to debunk them. Here are some myths that failed science class:

1. There's no evidence that taking a "birth control cleanse"—a supplement mix marketed to help a woman's body reset after stopping birth control—is legit. Since hormonal birth control can suppress the hormones released by the ovaries, it may take a few months (or not!) for a woman's cycle to naturally reset after stopping, but that's normal, and it doesn't mean you can't get pregnant during this time.

2. Sitting with your legs up is a great restorative yoga posture that increases circulation, but doing so after sex will not increase the chances of sperm fertilizing the egg. The fact is, sperm deposited at the cervix around ovulation are found in the fallopian tubes within 15 minutes,[5] and they don't need any help from gravity!

3. We won't stop you from pulling out the Kama Sutra, but there's no sex position that optimizes getting pregnant. Healthy sperm will find the egg, no matter what position you're in.

4. Some people also believe that peeing too quickly after sex can wash the sperm away, but there's no evidence to back this up. We suggest peeing fairly soon after sex to decrease your chances of getting a urinary tract infection.

5. Men should not worry that frequent ejaculation (from masturbation) will decrease their fertility.[6]

6. There's an urban myth that a woman's post-orgasm contractions "suck up" sperm and increase the chances of getting pregnant. Orgasms don't actually increase the likelihood of pregnancy. They're just fun.

7. You might especially want a girl or a boy, but that's up to mother nature—you can't time sex, or do any other of a number of old wives tales, to pick the sex of your future kid.

Putting The TLC in TTC

Trying to conceive (TTC) is a unique period in your life. Take advantage of this time to appreciate your body and its wondrous ability to create life by treating it the best you can.

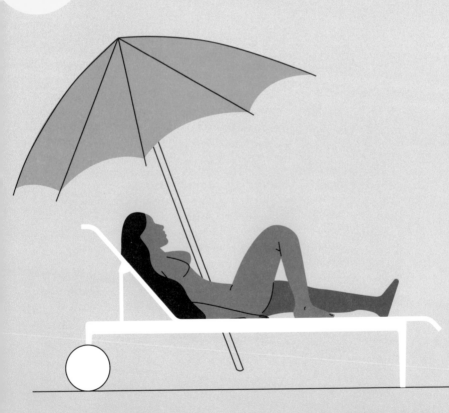

Lifestyle Factors and Fertility

Besides timing sex and tracking ovulation, there are general health and lifestyle factors that will influence your likelihood of getting pregnant and the health of a developing baby.[7] Now, more than ever, it's important to try and be aware of what you can do to practice good self care and mitigate risk by steering clear of known harmful substances.

Body weight | Women who are underweight (BMI <19) may take four times longer to get pregnant than women of average weight, while women who are obese (BMI > 30) may take twice as long.[8,9] Being overweight can also increase a woman's risk of developing pre-eclampsia, gestational diabetes, and complications during labor. There is conflicting data on whether or not obesity in men reduces fertility. Either way, if you're underweight or overweight, talk to your health provider or a nutritionist about making a plan.

Smoking | Smoking and secondhand exposure to smoke have major effects on fertility. It can delay conception and lead to higher rates of miscarriage.[10] Smoking may affect sperm function—but the research linking smoking with lower fertility in men isn't conclusive.[11] During pregnancy, tobacco use may also lead to fetal growth restriction, problems with the placenta that can lead to increased preterm birth, stillbirth, and premature rupture of the amniotic sac.

Caffeine | The data on how caffeine affects pregnancy is mixed. Most of the evidence doesn't show a link between caffeine usage and difficulty conceiving or miscarriage, but the American College of Obstetricians and Gynecologists (ACOG) and the March of Dimes recommend sticking to under 200 mg (one or two cups of coffee) per day.[12]

Medication | Some over-the-counter and prescription drugs can affect fertility. If you're trying to conceive, both partners should clear meds with their provider first.

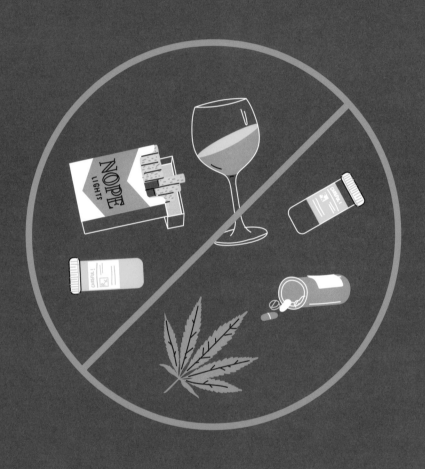

Alcohol	Excessive drinking may cause fertility problems, miscarriage, and a condition known as Fetal Alcohol Spectrum Disorder. We suggest eliminating alcohol consumption while trying to get pregnant. Drinking isn't great for male fertility either—in excess, it can reduce testosterone and decrease the production of sperm.[13]
Recreational or illegal drugs	Cocaine, meth, ecstasy, etc.—avoid them all. Just because weed is more readily available than ever doesn't mean it's safe to use in pregnancy. In animal models, THC (tetrahydrocannabinol, the part of marijuana responsible for its psychoactive effects) levels in the fetus were about 10% of what it was in maternal blood.[14] It's difficult to tease out the direct effects of marijuana in studies, but the data suggests a potential increase in premature labor or having an underweight baby.
Pollutants and toxins	Environmental pollutants and toxins, such as flame retardants and dry cleaning solvents, heavy metals like mercury and arsenic, pesticides, and possibly Bisphenol A (BPA) can have adverse effects on fertility and pregnancy.[15] It can be challenging to assess the degree and effect of exposure, and what to do to reduce exposure in some cases. Researchers are still studying the effects on reproductive health for some of these toxins.

Nutrition

Despite best efforts, it is hard to prepare your body for a healthy pregnancy through food alone, and it can be impossibly difficult for people with dietary restrictions or certain medical conditions. That's why it's highly recommended by ACOG that women planning a pregnancy take a complete prenatal vitamin.

The ideal time to start a prenatal vitamin routine is one to three months before trying to conceive. This allows you time to build up reserves of folate, which is important for its ability to prevent neural tube defects in the embryo's developing brain and spinal cord. You should continue to take your prenatal throughout the duration of your pregnancy, and possibly post-partum if you are breastfeeding.

A good prenatal vitamin should offer among many things:

Folate
Folate is instrumental in decreasing the risk of neural tube defects in the developing embryo. It's most effective when taken one to three months pre-pregnancy, so that you can build up adequate levels for critical developmental milestones in the first few weeks of growth.[16] It's so effective that the US government instituted mandatory food fortification programs of folic acid (a synthetic form of folate) in 1998.[17] A new form of folate used in dietary supplements, known as L-methylfolate (MTHF folate), is more easily used by the body (or *bioavailable*) and has less side effects than folic acid. Additionally, 25% of the population is severely impaired in their ability to use folic acid[16,18] and at an increased risk of having a child with neural tube defects.[18-20] The research is still preliminary, but these individuals may benefit from MTHF folate supplementation over folic acid as well.[16,21,22]

Iron
Your body uses iron to make hemoglobin, the protein that red blood cells use to transport oxygen. In your lungs, the hemoglobin in red blood cells binds to oxygen and carries it to all the tissues in your body, including a developing embryo via the placenta. The total amount of blood in a woman's body will increase by 50% during pregnancy,[23] so iron is in high demand. Iron supplements help to prevent pregnancy-induced anemia, a condition where you don't have enough hemoglobin in your blood.

Calcium
A growing baby needs calcium to build its bones and teeth, especially during the last three months of pregnancy. Breastfeeding also requires a lot of calcium from mom, with some studies showing that women can lose 3-5% of their bone mass during this time. This is a time where calcium is in high demand; supplementation ensures you have the nutrients you need. Calcium is best absorbed when it's paired with Vitamin D, so an ideal prenatal will have both.[24]

DHA
Also known as docosahexaenoic acid, DHA is an omega-3 fatty-acid. DHA is used to build the developing brain and eyes and is also important for long term cognitive and motor development.[25]

What to Look for in a Prenatal Vitamin

Supplements shouldn't replace a healthy diet, but instead ensure you're meeting the nutritional demands of pregnancy. ACOG recommends women take a prenatal vitamin one to three months before they begin trying to conceive.[23,24]

Look for a prenatal containing:

- 600 mcg of MTHF folate or folic acid
- 27 mg of iron
- 200-300 mg of DHA
- Vitamin D
- 1,000 mg calcium

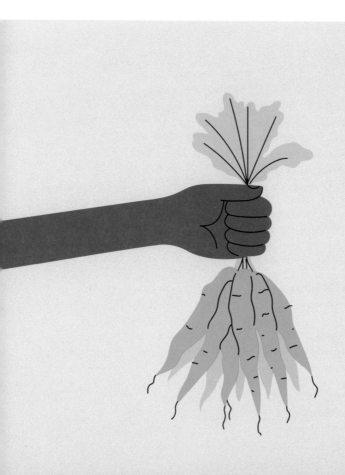

The Preconception Visit

A preconception visit with your healthcare provider is an important first step to pregnancy. The goal of the visit is to make sure you're healthy, prepared, and educated about what's ahead—including any risk factors for complications or needed lifestyle changes. It's also helpful to establish care with a provider and start developing a trusting relationship.

At your preconception visit your provider may bring up:

Reproductive history	Tell them about any previous pregnancies, sexually transmitted infections (STIs), pap smear results (make sure you're up-to-date on your cervical cancer screening!), menstrual history, and birth control use.
Medical history	It's important for your provider to know your comprehensive medical history to help determine potential risk factors and complications that may arise during pregnancy. If you're going into your pregnancy with conditions like asthma, diabetes, high blood pressure, depression, or thyroid disease, let your provider know. There are many medical conditions that have implications for pregnancy and should be discussed before conception. Make sure they have your medical records, and talk through your body's biography.
Past surgeries	Knowledge of past surgeries—big or small—helps your provider to understand your reaction to anesthesia and flag potential roadblocks in trying to conceive or deliver.
Family history	Your ethnicity, along with significant family history (like your sister who had pre-eclampsia or your aunt's gestational diabetes) can reveal things about your health. If possible, talk with your family before the visit to see if there's anything notable you should share.
Lifestyle	Keep it real. Tell your provider how often you exercise, how much you drink, etc.

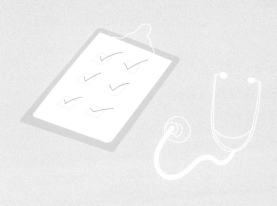

Medications	Tell your provider everything you're taking, even over-the-counter meds, vitamins, and supplements. Also mention things like retinol and salicylic acid— both are topical creams people use to combat acne that are not safe for pregnancy.
Genetic carrier screening	This is a test that parents can take to learn more about the genetic health of their future children. It looks to see if parents are carriers of any hidden genetic disorders that they may unknowingly pass on to their children. We'll talk more about this in the next section.
Domestic violence	Your preconception visit is a time to reflect on your relationship and make sure you feel emotionally and physically safe. If you feel unsafe, we urge you to speak with your provider. Intimate partner violence affects millions of women, irrespective of their age, socioeconomic status, race, or religion. Your provider can connect you with local resources and support.[28]
Travel plans	Talk to your provider to get the latest information about regions or countries to avoid concerns for certain infectious diseases, like the Zika virus.

Now is the time to talk openly with your provider. Consider practical questions ranging from how to use an ovulation test or find your fertile window to debunking the many myths we hear about medicine and wellness. Your provider is there to break it down and give you evidence-based advice. If you're feeling overwhelmed, your provider can also point you toward online resources, books, or counselors.

Genetic Carrier Screening

It's rare, but possible, for two completely healthy individuals to have a child with a life-threatening genetic disorder. Genetic carrier screening can help determine your family's risk of having a child with a genetic disorder. Genetic disorders are caused by the inheritance of defective genes (the building blocks of your DNA) from one or both parents. Screening can help identify these risk factors, even if you think you have nothing to pass on. Certain groups are known to have a higher risk of particular genetic conditions: for example, there's a higher prevalence of Tay-Sachs disease in Ashkenazi Jews, sickle cell anemia in African Americans, and blood disorders (thalassemias) in Southeast Asians and people of Mediterranean descent.[29-32] Consanguinity in your family tree (a marriage between cousins) increases the risk of having a child with a genetic disorder.

There are two types of screening tests:

Targeted carrier screening	In targeted screening you are tested for specific genetic disorders, usually based on your ethnicity and family history. Testing for cystic fibrosis alone would be an example of a targeted screen.
Expanded carrier screening	With expanded screening you are tested for many disorders using a single sample. These screens usually look at dozens or even hundreds of inherited genetic disorders. Some of the conditions tested are extremely rare and we still don't understand them well. It's important to discuss your results with a genetic counselor.

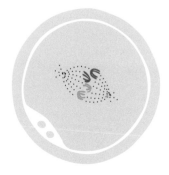
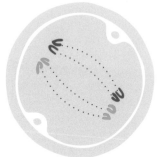

It may be nerve-wracking to undergo a test like this. Currently, ACOG recommends that couples trying to conceive receive targeted genetic carrier screening for two rare, but devastating, diseases: cystic fibrosis and spinal muscular atrophy.[29] The decision on whether or not to get an expanded carrier screening is a personal one that involves deciding what's important to you and what you would do with that information. Your provider can counsel you on whether it might be appropriate. If your preventive genetic testing comes back positive for a condition, talk to your provider about your options. If you know this information ahead of time, you may choose to use assistive reproductive technology to get pregnant with an embryo that doesn't carry the genetic disorder.

We want to acknowledge: this is a sticky, complicated area of discussion that needs to take into account your values and judgment. How important is it for you to know this information ahead of time? What will you do with the information if the results are positive or unclear? How will you feel if you're told you're a carrier for something that isn't life threatening, but can affect the quality of life of your future child? These are just a few of the questions that a genetic counselor can help you navigate.

The Journey to Pregnancy

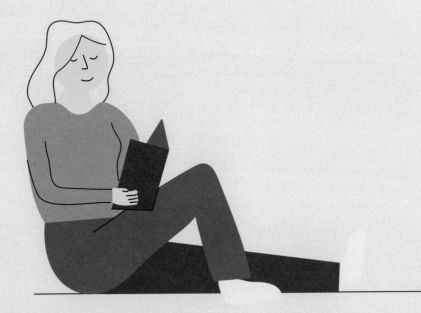

If you want to approach conception with the "knowledge is power" attitude, there are three main tools to use to get better at timing sex around the fertile window. In short, have lots of sex and have it as close to ovulation as possible.

Cervical Mucus

The cervical mucus test is a free and easy way for you to determine when ovulation is happening. Cervical mucus is the gooey discharge produced by the cervix. Its consistency and color changes in response to the body's monthly hormonal cycle and those changes can be used to determine the fertile window.

For women who want to do a cervical mucus test:

1. Begin recording the characteristics of your cervical mucus the day after your period stops. It's best to chart every day for your entire cycle to get to know the different characteristics.

2. Before you pee, insert a clean finger into your vagina to obtain a sample.

3. Take a look and note the color (yellow, white, clear, cloudy), amount (none, some, lots), consistency (thick, sticky, stretchy) and feel (dry, wet, or slippery).

The most common sign of the fertile window is when cervical mucus is abundant, stretchy, and clear, like a raw egg-white. (Figure 6) Sperm swim very quickly up the egg-white kind of cervical mucus,[33] improving the likelihood of conception.

Figure 6

Detecting Ovulation from Cervical Mucus

The texture of cervical mucus changes as you approach your fertile window. When you are in your fertile window, your cervical mucus resembles an egg-white in color and consistency.

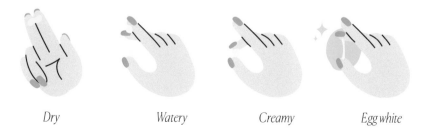

| *Dry* | *Watery* | *Creamy* | *Egg white* |

Fertile window

Ovulation Tests

You can also pinpoint your fertile window using ovulation tests (aka ovulation predictor kits or OPKs). The process is a lot like taking a pregnancy test because the test detects the presence of hormones in urine. Most ovulation tests try to identify when a woman is in an LH surge by detecting an abundance of LH in urine.[34,35] Remember, the brain releases this flood of LH to bring on ovulation, so if you can detect the presence of this surge, you can anticipate that ovulation will likely occur within 16 to 48 hours.[36] Figure 7 maps out when to begin using an ovulation test relative to day 1 of your cycle.

There are many types of ovulation tests—ones that you pee on directly, ones that have to be dipped into a cup of urine, ones that are digital—but they work by this same basic mechanism.

A note about using ovulation tests: if you have Polycystic Ovary Syndrome (PCOS), these may not be the best way to determine your fertile window. Women with PCOS may have consistently high levels of LH, leading them to get false positive results from ovulation tests (meaning the test will say they are ovulating when they are not). False positive results may also be elevated in women with irregular cycles.[37,38]

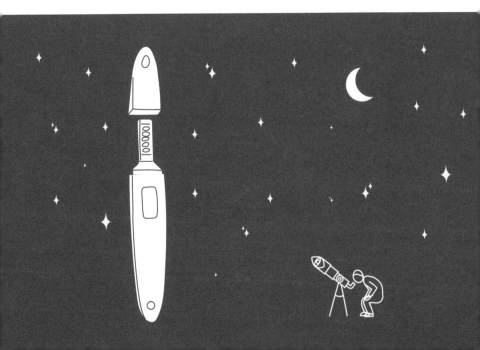

Figure 7

When to Use Ovulation Tests

Use this table to determine when to start using an ovulation test to find your fertile window. To figure out your cycle length, count the day your period starts (the first day of full menstrual flow) as day 1, and continue counting until the day before your next period starts. The total number of days is your cycle length. If your cycles are irregular, test based on the shortest cycle you've had in the last three months.

Cycle length in days	Day of cycle to start testing	Cycle length in days	Day of cycle to start testing
Less than 21 days	5	31	14
21	5	32	15
22	5	33	16
23	6	34	17
24	7	35	18
25	8	36	19
26	9	37	20
27	10	38	21
28	11	39	22
29	12	40	23
30	13	Over 40	17 days before next period

Basal Body Temperature

After you ovulate, your resting body temperature increases an almost imperceptible half a degree. You can detect this temperature change using an ultra-sensitive thermometer, called a basal body thermometer. This half a degree temperature rise confirms that ovulation has taken place.

But here's the catch: since a woman's body temperature increases in response to ovulation,[35,39] by the time you've detected this change it's too late to conceive in that cycle. If you have regular cycles, you can use that information to better know your cycle and help you predict when to have sex next month.

It can also be used to detect pregnancy—a rise in basal body temperature (BBT) that lasts for 18+ days may be an early indicator of pregnancy[2] (although by that time you'll probably already know from a pregnancy test!).

Here's how women can measure BBT to confirm ovulation:

1. Start recording your BBT on day one of your period. Your BBT from the first five days of your cycle will be used to determine your baseline temperature.

2. Place your thermometer on your bedside, within easy reach.

3. As soon as you wake up in the morning, but before you sit up, grab the thermometer and take your temperature under your tongue/arm.

4. Once you have a reading, record it in your chart.

5. Note your baseline BBT. Watch for an increase in temperature, which will typically be less than a half-degree Fahrenheit. This indicates you've ovulated. Once you have a higher temperature for three or more days, you can assume ovulation occurred.

This method is more laborious than the other two methods discussed for determining your fertile window. It's also more prone to error; interrupted sleep, jet lag, alcohol, illness, and even stress can influence BBT readings. That said, many women use BBT for cycle tracking. Choose the method that works best for you.

Testing for Pregnancy

Pregnancy tests can be either the most exciting or disappointing part of the TTC journey, depending on the result. Just like ovulation tests, there are many different types of pregnancy tests. All work by detecting human Chorionic Gonadotropin (hCG) in urine. hCG is the first detectable sign of pregnancy. It is produced by the embryo and placenta and can be detected in urine after the embryo implants itself into the uterine wall.

An important thing to know is when in your cycle you can take a pregnancy test. There are two types of pregnancy tests: "early-result" pregnancy tests (higher sensitivity tests) you can use before a missed period (ranging from one to six days before), and traditional pregnancy tests that are used after a missed period. Both of these can be either digital or analog (display a stripe for a positive result).

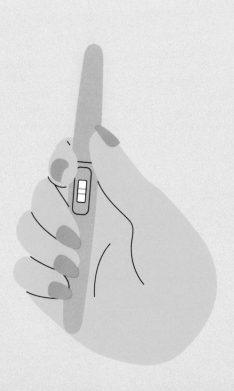

Generally, the closer you are to a potential missed period, the more accurate the results will be. Before your missed period, the embryo may not yet be implanted or producing enough hCG for the test to detect. The amount of hCG produced by the embryo ramps up quickly, essentially doubling every two days for the first four weeks of pregnancy,[2] so if you wait to test until close to your period, your results will be more conclusive.

No matter which type of test you use, emotions run high when the time comes to take a pregnancy test. Try to remember that the journey to conceive is a special time in your life, and to be gentle with yourself if the results do not turn out as you wish. We're crossing our fingers for you!

How Long it Takes

Hopefully you're now empowered with the information and tools you need to begin your conception journey. One last important thing to discuss is timing—how long does it take most couples to get pregnant?

In broad strokes, 92% of couples conceive within one year of trying, with the majority conceiving within six months (81%—Figure 8).[1] These odds are affected by age and other lifestyle factors discussed above, but this is a good benchmark to set expectations. If you're over 35, your statistics look very similar, but guidelines about when to seek the help of a fertility specialist are a little different.

Rules of thumb about when to seek the help of a reproductive endocrinologist and infertility specialist (REI) split at age 35:

- If you're *under* 35, doctors recommend trying for one year consistently before seeking the help of an REI.

- If you're *over* 35, doctors recommend trying for six months consistently before seeking the help of an REI.

If you don't conceive within six to 12 months, hang in there! You still have lots of options. We'll discuss them more in *Paths to Parenthood.*

Figure 8

Cumulative Probability of Pregnancy Over One Year

This data represents the probability of getting pregnant over a year of consistently trying to conceive for 346 women. The majority of women conceive within six months (81%). After one year, 92% of women are pregnant. This data is for all ages studied.

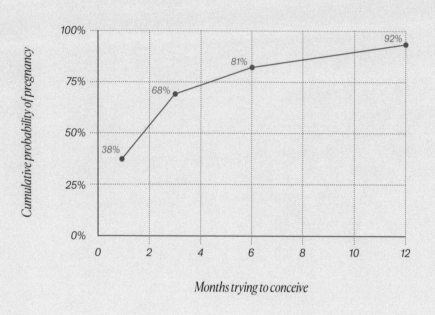

Adapted from Gnoth et al., 2003.[1]

Roadblocks

A few reproductive health conditions can make it more difficult to conceive. In fact, one in eight couples have trouble getting pregnant or sustaining a pregnancy.[40] If you've been diagnosed with any of the following, we encourage you to talk to an OBGYN or fertility specialist early on, before you start your TTC journey.

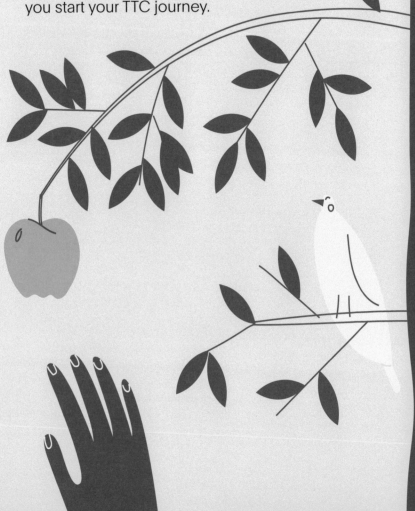

Female Factor

Conception is a complex process, and sometimes certain symptoms or other observable clinical signs allow your doctor to figure out which part of your body, or which of your body's processes, is causing infertility. These "factor" phrases are umbrella terms that allow clinicians to describe problems with that part or process, before they know exactly what's wrong within it. In women, doctors divide diagnoses into the following groups based on the part of the body that is responsible: endometrial or uterine factor, ovulatory dysfunction, tubal factor, cervical factor, and coital factor.

Uterine factor infertility describes abnormalities of the uterus that may make it more difficult to get pregnant:

Endometriosis	Endometriosis is a condition where the uterine lining (or endometrium) spreads outside of the uterus. It can grow on various parts of the pelvis: the ovaries, bladder, rectum—sometimes even under the diaphragm. That tissue is stimulated at the time of menses. Endometriosis can cause significant fertility issues because of the inflammatory reaction and often takes a long time to diagnose. It occurs in about one in ten women.[41] Symptoms during menstruation include ovarian cysts and severe pelvic pain during sex, urination, or bowel movements. If you're not trying to get pregnant, symptoms are treated with hormonal contraception. Your doctor may recommend surgery if there is concern for significant scarring.
Abnormal uterine anatomy	Abnormal uterine anatomy can impair embryo implantation and growth. Examples of such conditions include an abnormal shape to the uterus (septate uterus); uterine fibroids, non-cancerous, smooth muscle tumors that can make it difficult for an embryo to implant (think of it as an embryo trying to burrow itself into a cobblestone street); and intrauterine adhesions, scar tissue that grows in response to a prior uterine surgery (like a dilation and curettage).[42]

Ovulatory dysfunctions are responsible for 21% of all fertility issues:[41]

Polycystic Ovary Syndrome	PCOS is a hormone disorder affecting one in ten women that disrupts ovulation and can result in irregular periods. PCOS accounts for the vast majority of ovulatory disorders. Symptoms of PCOS include excess body hair, ovarian cysts (though not always, so it's a bit of a misnomer) and weight gain. PCOS can be treated with oral fertility drugs, IVF, and lifestyle-based interventions.[43,44]
Primary Ovarian Insufficiency	POI, formerly known as "premature ovarian failure," occurs when a woman's ovaries stop functioning before she is 40. POI (which is often mistakenly referred to as "premature menopause") accounts for 10-30% of ovulatory disorders. Onset is usually sudden. Some women may have an autoimmune or genetic condition that predisposes them to POI (though this is rare). Women with POI have very few to no periods, elevated FSH and LH, low estrogen, and experience hot flashes and vaginal dryness. It is still possible to conceive with POI, but may require extra support from your provider.[42]
Amenorrhea	Amenorrhea is the absence of menstruation. Women with amenorrhea are likely not ovulating. Amenorrhea can be caused by excessive stress, exercise, or low body weight. It accounts for only five to 10 percent of ovulatory disorders.[42]
Oligomen-orrhea from other causes	Oligomenorrhea is irregular or inconsistent periods. Sometimes the communication between ovarian hormones (progesterone and estrogen) and brain hormones (LH, FSH, prolactin and thyroid stimulating hormone) doesn't function as it should. This can result in irregular ovulation and periods, making it difficult to conceive.[42] Oligomenorrhea can be treated with oral fertility drugs.
Tubal factor	Tubal factor refers to a blockage of the fallopian tubes (the route the egg takes from the ovary to the uterus) and comprises 25-35% of female infertility.

Causes of tubal blockage include a history of abdominal surgeries that can cause adhesions or scarring, pelvic inflammatory disease (PID), and STIs like chlamydia.[42] Women with tubal factor infertility often have no noticeable symptoms and don't realize the problem until they try and fail to conceive. Sometimes, blockages can be treated by corrective surgery or a woman can pursue IVF.

Cervical factor

Cervical factor issues are related to cervical mucus, which helps transport sperm. Sometimes the body can't make enough cervical mucus because of cervical infections from PID or cervical scarring after surgery. Treatment of cervical factor issues may include placing semen directly into the uterus (a process called intrauterine insemination or IUI) or IVF.[42]

Coital factor

Also called coital failure. Some people have difficulty having sex, whether it's because of pain during intercourse (vaginismus), psychological barriers, difficulty with arousal, or a combination of all of the above. Depending on the cause, coital factor infertility can be treated using counseling, physical therapy, or IVF.

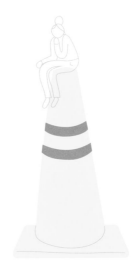

Male Factor

It's not all on women to carry the fertility torch. The burden of infertility is shared pretty equally among men and women: roughly a third is attributed to women alone, a third is attributed to men alone, and the remaining third is attributed to a combination of the two.[41]

In the cases where male-factors are to blame, they generally fall into four groups:[45,46]

1. Azoospermia: no sperm present in semen

2. Oligospermia: low sperm count

3. Asthenospermia: low sperm motility or "slow swimmers"

4. Teratozoospermia: abnormal sperm shape or morphology

The underlying causes of these sperm abnormalities isn't always known. One potential cause is varicocele, which is the enlargement of the scrotal veins. Varicocele affects approximately 40% of infertile men.[45,47] It can be repaired using surgical methods, depending on the severity and location of the varicocele. Lifestyle improvements, such as maintaining a healthy BMI, getting enough sleep, and drinking in moderation can also improve sperm health.[13,48] Additionally, IUI or IVF with intracytoplasmic sperm injection (ICSI), a technique where a single sperm is injected directly into an egg to form an embryo, may be used as treatment.[46]

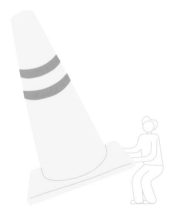

Unexplained infertility

Finally, as much as our knowledge and ability to troubleshoot fertility has advanced in the last few decades, there's still a lot we don't know. For about 15% to 30% of infertile couples, clinicians will fail to determine the exact cause of infertility.[41] If this is you, there is still hope; after trying unsuccessfully for 12 months, 50% of couples with unexplained infertility get pregnant within the next 12 months, and another 12% get pregnant the following year.[49]

While this is an exciting journey, it has its difficulties. If you feel like you need more support outside the provider's office, we recommend seeking the help of a mental health provider. Support groups (online and offline) are also a great way to find support by connecting with peers facing similar challenges.

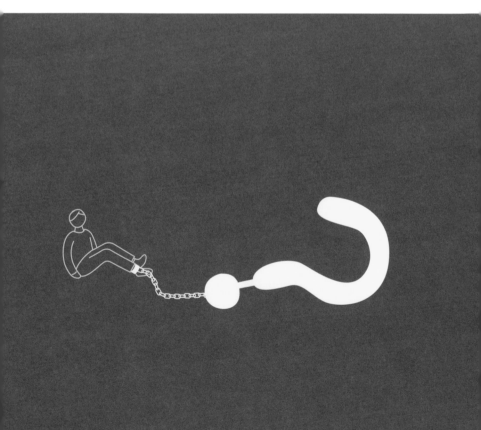

Miscarriage

While medical advances have come a very long way, miscarriages still happen to about three million women every year in the United States. A miscarriage is a loss in the first 20 weeks of pregnancy, and is most common during the first trimester: around 80% of miscarriages happen during the first 13 weeks of pregnancy.[2]

The cause of a miscarriage isn't always clear, but they're thought to most commonly result from the embryo's chromosomal abnormalities. Overall, the risk of miscarriage from a single pregnancy is approximately 14%.[50] Age is a significant factor in determining your risk for miscarriage: there is a steep climb in the rate of miscarriages right at age 35 (Figure 9). This statistic underlies the dreaded reduction in fertility at age 35.[50] If you're concerned about miscarriage, talk with your provider.

Everyone feels differently about when and to whom they should share the news of their pregnancy. Some wait until after the risk of miscarriage goes down (after the first trimester). On the other hand, if you experience a pregnancy loss, grieving alone can be lonely and painful. Although it may be hard to appreciate this at the time, the silver lining of miscarriage, especially in couples battling infertility, is that you were able to conceive. Do what's best for you and your partner. If you need help after pregnancy loss, consider talking with a mental health counselor or your family and close friends. Remember, miscarriages are more common than you would expect from public discussion—it's likely you will find an understanding shoulder to lean (or cry) on if you open up.

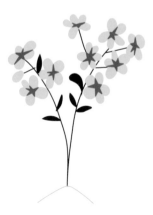

Figure 9

Miscarriage Rate by Age of the Mother

Women are more likely to miscarry as they age, with a steep rise starting at age 35.

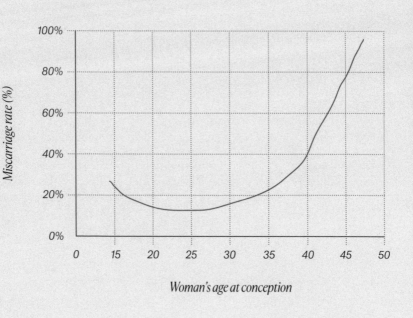

Woman's age at conception

Adapted from Anderson et. al, 2000.[50]

Paths to Parenthood

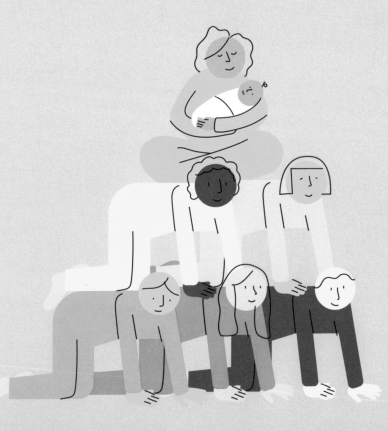

If you're struggling to conceive naturally, there are many other paths to parenthood. Modern medicine can lend a helping hand when our inborn biology lets us down. Here are some additional paths:

- Oral fertility drugs, such as Clomid and Letrozole, regulate or stimulate ovulation. This is the most common first path of treatment for women who struggle to get pregnant due to ovulation disorders. While taking these drugs, you'd still try to conceive naturally. These medications help to ensure your body releases an egg at the right time. One caveat is that Clomid can increase your risk of multiples (e.g. twins).[51]

- Intrauterine insemination (IUI) is a fertility treatment that places sperm directly inside the uterus using a catheter. The procedure is relatively fast and painless, which is why many people choose to do multiple rounds of IUI before moving onto IVF.[51]

- IVF takes the fertilization part of the operation out of your hands. Egg and sperm are isolated from both parents and fertilized outside of the body (in-vitro). To isolate eggs, a woman takes hormones that hyper-stimulate her ovaries to mature many eggs at once. These eggs are then retrieved under anesthesia. The father then contributes sperm (in a much simpler "procedure"). The eggs are then fertilized in a lab and implanted in the uterus, with the rest of the pregnancy proceeding naturally. This entire process is considered one cycle of IVF. IVF is an incredible technology, and it's helped many people get pregnant.
Just keep in mind that it can be a long, trying process. The medication required to mature multiple eggs and the procedure to retrieve them can be difficult and painful. IVF can also take a few cycles to work, which is a hassle, because it requires you to be on a pretty intensive schedule, including a lot of doctor appointments. It's also not always covered by insurance—and if it's not covered, it's very expensive.[52,53]

There are other alternative paths to pregnancy, too. There's the possibility of donation-assisted pregnancy, with either donor eggs or donor sperm. The donation can be done through a service agency, or with a friend or family member who offers to help. With the advent of consumer genetic tests, just don't expect anonymity in the donor process anymore.

For those who are unable to carry a child (for biological or medical reasons), a gestational carrier (GC) or surrogate is another option. A GC carries the pregnancy for a person or couple unable to on their own. GCs are not biologically related to the child unless they are a family member, or the egg donor.

Finally, there are paths to parenthood beyond pregnancy that are equally exciting. Fostering and/or adoption is beautiful way to build a family. There are over 600,000 children in foster care and over 135,000 children adopted in the United States each year. Of US-based adoptions, 59% are from the foster system, 26% are international adoptions, and 15% are other American adoptions.[54] Requirements for fostering and adoption vary based on state or country. Check out the National Council for Adoption for more info.

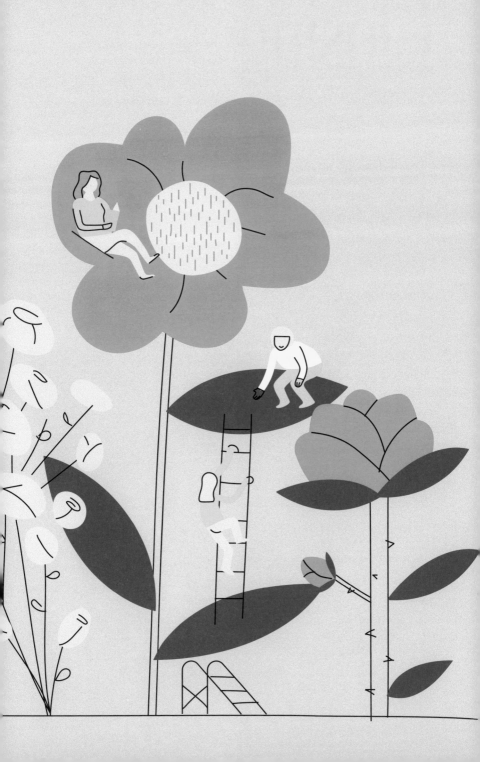

Closing

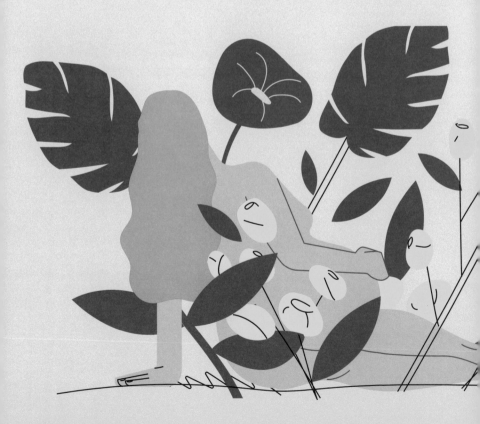

We hope this book has empowered you with the tools and knowledge you need to start your journey into parenthood. We're excited for you as you start this new chapter of your life! We hope you'll look back at the sections of this book as you need them. But most of all, we hope you find levity, happiness, and strength through this wild ride.

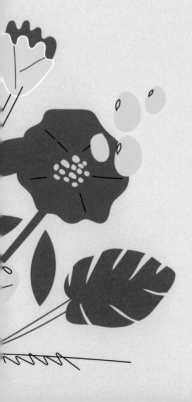

Glossary

Amenorrhea	Lack of periods.
ACOG	American College of Obstetrics and Gynecology. A professional association of obstetricians and gynecologists.
Assisted reproductive technology (ART)	Medical procedures to treat infertility that combine sperm and egg outside of the body. IVF is an example of ART.
Asthenospermia	The medical diagnosis of a man whose sperm swim relatively slowly (reduced motility).
Azoospermia	The medical diagnosis of a man whose semen contains no sperm.
Basal body temperature (BBT)	A woman's resting body temperature. It rises approximately half a degree in response to ovulation.
Bioavailability	A measure of how easily a drug can be utilized by the body.
Body Mass Index (BMI)	A measurement of body fat based on the ratio of weight to height.
Calcium	A mineral that is essential for building bones and teeth in the developing fetus.
Cervical Mucus	Mucus produced by the cervix. Its characteristics change throughout the menstrual cycle and can indicate when a woman is in her fertile window.
Cervix	The opening to the uterus. Sperm must pass through the cervix and uterus to reach an egg.
Conception	The moment a sperm fertilizes an egg.
Corpus luteum	A progesterone producing structure located within the ovaries that forms from the follicle that releases an egg.
Dilation and curettage (D&C)	A medical procedure to remove tissue from inside the uterus. A D&C can be performed to diagnose and treat uterine conditions, to clear the uterus of pregnancy tissue after a miscarriage, or during an abortion.
Docosahexaenoic Acid (DHA)	An omega-3 fatty acid that is important for brain and eye development. It can be found in fatty fish or omega-3 supplemented dairy and eggs.
Egg	The female reproductive cells produced in the ovaries. Also known as the ovum.

Embryo	An early stage of human development. When an egg is fertilized, an embryo is created. It then grows, matures, and develops until it reaches a developmental milestone at 11 weeks gestation, when it becomes a fetus.
Endometriosis	A condition where the endometrium (inner cells of the uterus) grow outside the uterus. Endometriosis can affect fertility and cause painful periods.
Endometrium	The inner lining of the uterus. This layer thickens and sheds during menstruation. It is also the layer of the uterus where an embryo will implant.
Estrogen	The primary sex hormone in women, mainly produced by the ovaries (follicles) and placenta. It helps to regulate the menstrual cycle. It is also present in men, controlling libido, sperm production, and other important sexual functions.
Fallopian tube	The two tubes connecting the ovaries to the uterus, where sperm fertilize the egg. The tubes have little hairs inside (cilia) to help the egg travel from the ovary to the uterus.
Fertile window	The time when a woman is most likely to conceive. It is the six days preceding and including the day of ovulation.
Fertilization	The process by which a sperm and egg combine to form an embryo. During natural conception, this occurs in the fallopian tube.
Folate	A B vitamin (B9) known to decrease the risk of neural tube defects. It refers to the class of folates found in foods and dietary supplements. This includes folic acid and MTHF folate.
Folic acid	A synthetic form of folate used in food fortification programs in the US and found in prenatal vitamins. It is most effective at lowering the risk of neural tube defects in a developing embryo when taken one to three months before conception.
Follicle Stimulating Hormone (FSH)	A hormone produced in the brain that helps coordinate the menstrual cycle. It promotes the maturation of immature eggs inside the ovary.
Follicular phase	The first half of the menstrual cycle, from the onset of menstruation until ovulation.
Gene	The building blocks of our DNA. They are passed from parent to child.

Genetic carrier screening	A type of genetic testing done on parents, usually before they try to conceive, to identify risk factors for genetic disorders. These include spinal muscular atrophy and cystic fibrosis, among others.
Genetic disorder	A disease resulting from a genetic mutation. Cystic fibrosis and spinal muscular atrophy are both genetic disorders.
Gestational carrier (GC)	Also known as a surrogate, a GC is a woman who carries a pregnancy for a couple who is unable to on their own. A GC usually does not have any genetic relation to the child she carries.
Hemoglobin	The protein within red blood cells that binds oxygen and carries it throughout your body.
Human Chorionic Gonadotropin (hCG)	A hormone made by the early embryo or placenta, hCG is the first detectable sign of pregnancy. hCG is what is detected by home pregnancy tests.
Implantation	The process by which an embryo buries itself into the uterine wall. This usually occurs nine days after ovulation.[3]
In-vitro fertilization (IVF)	IVF is the process of combining a sperm and egg outside of the body to treat infertility. IVF is a type of ART.
Infertility	Inability to conceive after 12 months of unprotected sex.
Intracytoplasmic sperm injection (ICSI)	Fertilizing an egg by injecting a single sperm directly inside it.
Intrauterine Insemination (IUI)	A fertility intervention where sperm is deposited directly into the uterus.
Iron	A mineral that is an essential component of hemoglobin.
L-methylfolate (MTHF) folate	The active form of folate that your body uses. It is found in newer dietary supplements. It is most effective at lowering the risk of neural tube defects in a developing embryo when taken one to three months before conception.
LH surge	The steep rise in Lutenizing Hormone that precedes ovulation. This surge is detected by ovulation tests to identify a woman's fertile window.

Luteal phase	The second half of the menstrual cycle, from ovulation until the onset of the next menstrual cycle. The active form of folate that your body uses. It is found in newer dietary supplements. It is most effective at lowering the risk of neural tube defects in a developing embryo when taken one to three months before conception.
Luteinizing Hormone (LH)	A hormone produced in the brain that coordinates the menstrual cycle and induces ovulation.
Menopause	The cessation of menstrual periods.
Menstrual cycle	Cyclical changes in the female reproductive system that allow for pregnancy. This includes the building and shedding of the uterine lining, egg maturation, and ovulation, followed by either embryo implantation (if pregnancy occurs) or menstruation (if pregnancy does not occur). On average, this is 28 days.
Menstruation	The cyclical shedding of the uterine lining, commonly known as a period.
Miscarriage	A pregnancy loss that occurs before 20 weeks.
Neural-tube	The embryonic precursor to the brain and spinal cord.
Neural-tube defects	Developmental defects of the neural tube. These include spina bifida and anencephaly (the two most common types of neural tube defects). The incidence in the United States of these two types is 5.5 to 6.5 per 10,000 births.[50]
OBGYN	Abbreviation for the medical specialties of obstetrics and gynecology. Obstetrics covers pregnancy, childbirth, and the post-partum period. Gynecology covers the health of the female reproductive system.
Oligomenorrhea	Infrequent or irregular periods.
Oligospermia	The medical diagnosis of a man with low sperm count.
Ovarian follicle	The fluid filled sac in the ovary that contains an egg and its associated support cells.
Ovaries	The female sex organs. Equivalent to the male testes. Most women have two. They produce eggs (in a process known as oogenesis) and are connected to the uterus via the fallopian tubes.

Ovulation	The release of a mature egg from an ovary. Usually occurs around day 14 of the menstrual cycle.
Ovulation Test	At-home tests that detect when a woman is in her LH surge to identify her fertile window. Also known as ovulation predictor kits (OPKs).
Polycystic Ovary Syndrome (PCOS)	A hormonal disorder marked by irregular or absent menstrual periods, ovarian cysts, excess body hair, and difficulty getting pregnant.
Post-partum	The period after childbirth.
Pregnancy induced anemia	A condition brought on by pregnancy when blood does not have enough hemoglobin.
Pregnancy test	At-home tests that determine if a woman is pregnant by detecting the presence of hCG in a woman's urine.
Prenatal	Before or during pregnancy.
Prenatal vitamins	Vitamins designed to be taken before, during, and after pregnancy to ensure that a pregnant woman is receiving enough nutrients to support her and a developing child.
Primary Ovarian Insufficiency (POI)	The loss of ovarian function before age 40.
Progesterone	A female sex hormone produced by the ovaries (corpus luteum), adrenal glands, and placenta. It regulates the menstrual cycle and supports a pregnancy.
Puberty	The onset and development of the capability of sexual reproduction.
Semen	Fluid that contains sperm.
Sexually Transmitted Infections (STIs)	Also referred to as sexually transmitted diseases, STIs are infections spread by sex. They include chlamydia, herpes, gonorrhea, syphilis, HIV/AIDS, etc.
Sperm	The male reproductive cell produced in the testes.
TTC	A commonly used acronym for the phrase "trying to conceive."
Teratozoospermia	The medical diagnosis of a man with abnormally shaped sperm.
Testes	The male reproductive organs. Equivalent to the female ovaries. They produce sperm.

Testosterone	A male sex hormone. It is produced mainly by the testes. In men, it regulates sperm production, sexual arousal, the development of sexual reproduction, muscle development, and behavior. In women, testosterone helps to maintain bone mass and regulate sexual arousal.
Tetrahydrocannabinol (THC)	The component of marijuana that makes you feel high (psychoactive).
Two week wait (TWW)	The two weeks between ovulation and when you can take a pregnancy test.
Uterus	Also known as a womb, this is where an embryo will develop during pregnancy. It is connected to the ovaries via the fallopian tubes. If you're not pregnant, the lining (endometrium) sheds as your period.
Varicocele	The enlargement of a vein in the scrotum.

References

1   Gnoth, C., Godehardt, D., Godehardt, E., Frank-Herrmann, P. & Freundl,
        G. Time to pregnancy: results of the German prospective study and
        impact on the management of infertility. Hum. Reprod. 18, 1959–1966
        (2003).

2   Jones, R. E. & Lopez, K. H. Human reproductive biology: Third edition.
        (2006).

3   Wilcox, A. J., Baird, D. D. & Weinberg, C. R. Time of implantation of the
        conceptus and loss of pregnancy. N. Engl. J. Med. 340, 1796–1799
        (1999).

4   Practice Committee of American Society for Reproductive Medicine
        in collaboration with Society for Reproductive Endocrinology and
        Infertility. Optimizing natural fertility. Fertil. Steril. 90, S1–6 (2008).

5
        Ahlgren, M. Sperm transport to and survival in the human fallopian tube.
        Gynecol. Invest. 6, 206–214 (1975).

6   Mayorga-Torres, B. J. M. et al. Influence of ejaculation frequency on
        seminal parameters. Reprod. Biol. Endocrinol. 13, (2015).

7   Hassan, M. A. M. & Killick, S. R. Negative lifestyle is associated with a
        significant reduction in fecundity. Fertil. Steril. 81, 384–392 (2004).

8   Luke, B. et al. The effect of increasing obesity on the response to and
        outcome of assisted reproductive technology: a national study. Fertil.
        Steril. 96, 820–825 (2011).

9   Meldrum, D. R. Introduction: Obesity and reproduction. Fertil. Steril. 107,
        831–832 (2017).

10   Hyland, A. et al. Associations between lifetime tobacco exposure with
        infertility and age at natural menopause: the Women's Health Initiative
        Observational Study. Tob. Control 25, 706–714 (2016).

11   Penzias, A. et al. Smoking and infertility: a committee opinion. Fertil.
        Steril. 110, 611–618 (09/2018).

12   American College of Obstetrics and Gynecologists. Moderate Caffeine
        Consumption During Pregnancy. (2010).

13   Ricci, E. et al. Semen quality and alcohol intake: a systematic review
        and meta-analysis. Reprod. Biomed. Online 34, 38–47 (2017).

14   Conner, S. N. et al. Maternal Marijuana Use and Adverse Neonatal
        Outcomes: A Systematic Review and Meta-analysis. Obstet. Gynecol.
        128, 713–723 (10/2016).

15   Resources: Info For Families | Program on Reproductive Health and the
        Environment. Program on Reproductive Health and the Environment
        Available at: https://prhe.ucsf.edu/info. (Accessed: July 2019)

16   Greenberg, J. A., Bell, S. J., Guan, Y. & Yu, Y.-H. Folic Acid
        supplementation and pregnancy: more than just neural tube defect
        prevention. Rev. Obstet. Gynecol. 4, 52–59 (2011).

17   Mills, J. L. & Signore, C. Neural tube defect rates before and after food
        fortification with folic acid. Birth Defects Res. A Clin. Mol. Teratol. 70,
        844–845 (2004).

18   Liew, S.-C. & Gupta, E. D. Methylenetetrahydrofolate reductase (MTHFR)
        C677T polymorphism: Epidemiology, metabolism and the associated
        diseases. Eur. J. Med. Genet. 58, 1–10 (2015).

19   de Franchis, R. et al. The C677T mutation of the
        5,10-methylenetetrahydrofolate reductase gene is a moderate risk
        factor for spina bifida in Italy. J. Med. Genet. 35, 1009–1013 (1998).

20   Pietrzik, K., Bailey, L. & Shane, B. Folic Acid and L-5-
        Methyltetrahydrofolate. Clin. Pharmacokinet. 49, 535–548 (2010).

21   Obeid, R., Holzgreve, W. & Pietrzik, K. Is 5-methyltetrahydrofolate an
        alternative to folic acid for the prevention of neural tube defects? J.
        Perinat. Med. 41, 469–483 (2013).

22   Scaglione, F. & Panzavolta, G. Folate, folic acid and
        5-methyltetrahydrofolate are not the same thing. Xenobiotica 44,
        480–488 (2014).

23   Soma-Pillay, P. et al. Physiological changes in pregnancy. Cardiovasc. J.
        Afr. 27, 89–94 (2016).

24   Prentice, A. Maternal calcium requirements during pregnancy and
        lactation. Am. J. Clin. Nutr. 59, 477S–482S; discussion 482S–483S
        (1994).

25   Braarud, H. C. et al. Maternal DHA Status during Pregnancy Has a
        Positive Impact on Infant Problem Solving: A Norwegian Prospective
        Observation Study. Nutrients 10, (2018).

26   Kominiarek, M. A. & Rajan, P. Nutrition Recommendations in Pregnancy
        and Lactation. Med. Clin. North Am. 100, 1199–1215 (2016).

27   Williams, D. J. Nutrition in pregnancy. Oxford Medicine Online (2010).
        doi:10.1093/med/9780199204854.003.1402

28   American College of Obstetricians and Gynecologists. Intimate partner
        violence. (Obstet Gynecol , 2012).

29   Carrier Screening for Genetic Conditions - ACOG. Available at: https://
        www.acog.org/Clinical-Guidance-and-Publications/Committee-
        Opinions/Committee-on-Genetics/Carrier-Screening-for-Genetic-
        Conditions?IsMobileSet=false. (Accessed: July 2019)

30   Su, Y.-N. et al. Carrier Screening for Spinal Muscular Atrophy (SMA) in
        107,611 Pregnant Women during the Period 2005–2009: A Prospective
        Population-Based Cohort Study. PLoS One 6, e17067–e17067 (2011).

31   Strom, C. M. et al. Cystic fibrosis testing 8 years on: Lessons learned
        from carrier screening and sequencing analysis. Genet. Med. 13,
        166–172 (2011).

32   Naik, R. P. & Haywood, C., Jr. Sickle cell trait diagnosis: clinical and
        social implications. Hematology Am. Soc. Hematol. Educ. Program
        2015, 160–167 (2015).

33   Wallach, E. & Blasco, L. Clinical Approach to the Evaluation of Sperm-
        Cervical Mucus Interactions**Supported by Contract N01-HD-4-2838
        from the National Institutes of Health. Fertil. Steril. 28, 1133–1145 (11/1977).

34   Eichner, S. F. & Timpe, E. M. Urinary-Based Ovulation and Pregnancy:
        Point-of-Care Testing. Ann. Pharmacother. 38, 325–331 (02/2004).

35   Su, H., Yi, Y., Wei, T., Chang, T. & Cheng, C. Detection of ovulation, a
        review of currently available methods. Bioengineering & Translational
        Medicine 2, 238–238 (2017).

36   Leiva, R. A., Bouchard, T. P., Abdullah, S. H. & Ecochard, R. Urinary
        Luteinizing Hormone Tests: Which Concentration Threshold Best
        Predicts Ovulation? Front. Public Health 5, 320 (2017).

37   McGovern, P. G. et al. Absence of secretory endometrium after false-
        positive home urine luteinizing hormone testing. Fertil. Steril. 82,
        1273–1277 (2004).

38   Lloyd, R. & Coulam, C. B. The accuracy of urinary luteinizing hormone
        testing in predicting ovulation. Am. J. Obstet. Gynecol. 160, 1370–1375
        (6/1989).

39   Moghissi, K. S. Accuracy of Basal Body Temperature for Ovulation
        Detection**Presented at the Thirty-Second Annual Meeting of The
        American Fertility Society, April 5 to 9, 1976, Las Vegas, Nev. Fertil. Steril.
        27, 1415–1421 (1976).

40   2006-2010 National Survey For Family Growth - CDC. (2019). Available
        at: https://www.cdc.gov/nchs/nsfg/nsfg_2006_2010_puf.htm.
        (Accessed: July 2019)

41   Hull, M. G. et al. Population study of causes, treatment, and outcome of
        infertility. Br. Med. J. 291, 1693–1697 (1985).

42   Kuohung, W., Hornstein, M. D. & Levine, D. Evaluation of female infertility.
        UpToDate (2019). Available at: https://www.uptodate.com/contents/
        evaluation-of-female-infertility/print?search=diagnosis. (Accessed: July
        2019)

43   Teede, H., Deeks, A. & Moran, L. Open Access REVIEW Polycystic ovary
        syndrome: a complex condition with psychological, reproductive and
        metabolic manifestations that impacts on health across the lifespan.
        41–41 (2010).

44   Barbieri, R. L. & Ehrmann, D. A. Treatment of polycystic ovary syndrome
        in adults. (2019). Available at: https://www.uptodate.com/contents/
        treatment-of-polycystic-ovary-syndrome-in-adults. (Accessed: July
        2019)

45   Anawalt, B. D. & Page, S. T. Causes of Male Infertility. UpToDate (2019).
        Available at: https://www.uptodate.com/contents/causes-of-male-
        infertility. (Accessed: July 2019)

46   Anawalt, B. D. & Page, S. T. Treatments for male infertility. (2017).
        Available at: https://www.uptodate.com/contents/treatments-for-male-
        infertility. (Accessed: July 2019)

47   Practice Committee of the American Society for Reproductive Medicine
        & Society for Male Reproduction and Urology. Report on varicocele and
        infertility: a committee opinion. Fertil. Steril. 102, 1556–1560 (2014).

48   Campagne, D. M. Can Male Fertility Be Improved Prior to Assisted
        Reproduction through The Control of Uncommonly Considered
        Factors? Int J Fertil Steril 6, 214–223 (2013).

49   Gelbaya, T. A., Potdar, N., Jeve, Y. B. & Nardo, L. G. Definition and
        epidemiology of unexplained infertility. Obstet. Gynecol. Surv. 69,
        109–115 (2014).

50   Andersen, A.-M. N., Wohlfahrt, J., Christens, P., Olsen, J. & Melbye, M.
        Maternal age and fetal loss: population based register linkage study.
        BMJ 320, 1708–1712 (2000).

51   Kuohung, W. Treatments for female infertility. UpToDate (2019). Available
        at: https://www.uptodate.com/contents/treatments-for-female-
        infertility. (Accessed: July 2019)

52   Kessler, L. M., Craig, B. M., Plosker, S. M., Reed, D. R. & Quinn, G. P.
        Infertility Evaluation and Treatment among Women in the United States.
        Fertil. Steril. 100, (2013).

53   Katz, P. et al. Costs of infertility treatment: results from an 18-month
        prospective cohort study. Fertil. Steril. 95, 915–921 (2011).

54   POV. Fact Sheet | Off and Running | POV | PBS. POV | American
        Documentary Inc. (2010). Available at: http://archive.pov.org/
        offandrunning/fact-sheet. (Accessed: July 2019)

55   Williams, J. et al. Updated estimates of neural tube defects prevented
        by mandatory folic Acid fortification - United States, 1995-2011. MMWR
        Morb. Mortal. Wkly. Rep. 64, 1–5 (2015).